I0416061

The Effectiveness of Leadership in the Stop Smoking Campaign

Jennifer M. Valentine

ISBN-13: 978-1492213710
ISBN-10: 1492213713

DEDICATION:

To the NHS and our local Fire Brigade services

CONTENTS

FOREWORD

Like all good stop smoking books my aim in this publication is to highlight the passion behind the walk-in clinics, provide convincing testimonies, as well as mentioning the alternative to smoking tobacco – "electronic cigarettes." In this cigarette the liquid used contains nicotine, vegetable glycerine and propylene glycol compared to the approximately 600 different and damaging ingredients found in normal cigarettes. Effective leadership will establish a clear vision. They will share their vision with others so that they will follow willingly and then provide the information, knowledge and methods to realise that vision. The main problem that leaders of our young people have today is trying to convince them that marijuana is not a safer alternative to using tobacco. Their concern is that this activity or lifestyle contributes to a challenging life and even an early death.

Patty Baker from Teen Challenge USA wrote in 2012 about teens who regularly smoke marijuana: "they are putting themselves at risk of permanently damaging their intelligence as adults and are also significantly more likely to have attention and memory problems later in life, than their peers who abstained, according to a new study conducted by Duke University and London's King's College. This study is among the first to distinguish between cognitive problems the person might have had before using marijuana, and those that were caused by the drug." Patty went on to say that the research found that adults who started smoking pot as teenagers and used it heavily, but quit as adults, did not regain their full mental powers. In fact, persistent users who started as teenagers suffered a drop of eight IQ points at the age of 38, compared to when they were thirteen.

INTRODUCTION

Smoking starts off as a desire to emulate those around us. Influence is always the main reason for starting a journey. How long this journey goes on depends upon how settled and content one is with continuing. Smoking will soon become an addictive habit unless "number one" decides that this activity and its craving is no longer essential. As well as clinicians, theorists, and local authorities, the Department of Health still continues to prove that the leadership behind the ongoing Stop Smoking campaign is an effective one. Why should you or I be interested in that fact? Well, smoking pollutes our environment, turns a passive individual into a person at risk, not forgetting that it contributes to over 1000 cancer related diagnosis a year. Over the years the act of smoking has been challenged and even put into touch, especially by restaurants owners and publicans. Most cigarettes are now wrapped in plain packaging. The media no longer views smoking as a fashion accessory; it is now the "grim reaper." The price of cigarettes has risen considerably over the years so to say that smoking is the only affordable form of comfort is now a myth. My role is to work towards and provide good options for good health provided by a good service. I offer my time freely towards a voluntary position that requires full time training lead by a qualified stop smoking practitioner.

How does effective leadership take shape within the No Smoking Campaign? Firstly, there are Walk-In clinics and advisors located within every local authority.

The NHS leader's vision and aim is to improve quality, possess the ability to deliver and to provide high quality care. Their hope is that their managers are able to work in partnership with this vision too. Herman (2005) said that "managers make practical and strategic choices that give precedence to fulfilling the mission of the organisation." The effectiveness of leadership in the stop smoking campaign will depend on the objectives of the Department of Health. I am content to rely upon Handy's (1993) book which expressed that "objectives are to benefit the organisations expectations for success." The aim of the Department of Health is to inform the public about the dangers of smoking. These areas are made evident by means of a public health literature, the five stage programme (which every smoker must go through to stop smoking), and there are the effective advertising campaigns and outreach programmes. The public health practitioners are the ones who bring life to the path that leads towards reaching an effective success.

During the Conservative administration of 1979-1997 author Goodwin (2006) remarked that the Labour government concluded that "the failure of the NHS management to deliver a comprehensive and consumer sensitive NHS, reflected a failure of leadership in the NHS." Paul Edmondson-Jones, director of public health and primary care for NHS Portsmouth and Portsmouth city council, points out that better public health saves money and that not improving it is extremely costly because of "the financial pressures, the NHS may disinvest from some public health work in preventive services to make short-term gains." He went on to say, "smoking, obesity and alcohol place a massive burden on the NHS. Each of those can take ten years off your life expectancy." How does effective leadership take shape within the No Smoking Campaign? Within the NHS the leader's vision and aim is to improve quality, possess the ability to deliver and to provide high quality care. Their hope is that their managers are able to work in partnership with this vision too. Author Herman (2005) said that "managers make practical and strategic choices that give precedence to fulfilling the mission of the organisation." The effectiveness of leadership in the stop smoking campaign will depend on the objectives of the Department of Health which is to inform the public the dangers of smoking. These objectives are made evident by means of public health literature, the five stage programme (which every investigating smoker must go through), and effective advertising campaigns and outreach programmes. The public health practitioners are the ones who bring life to the path that leads towards reaching an effective success.

1 EFFECTIVE TARGETS

Each local authority set local targets for NHS Stop Smoking services. All smokers will have a cessation date of three months. Leaders will also give advice on managing cravings and how the free Local NHS Stop Smoking services can help an individual create their own plan to quit. There may be a need to question an individual's ethical beliefs by asking them if they are aware of the dangers passed on to others from second-hand smoking (i.e. smoke that is breathed back out by smokers). By focusing on the descriptive rather than a normative, the NHS Stop Smoking service is able to lead effectively within the local community. Once a patient or client is identified as being a smoker, information will be provided about stop smoking services. There then follows and initial motivation and assessment appointment. The required support will be agreed by:

a. Offering a weekly stop smoking programme for a minimum of five weeks.

b. Giving advice on and providing a twelve week programme of medication namely NRT, Champix or Zyban.

c. Offering one to one or group specialist advice.

d. Referring smokers to the specialist Level III service, particularly the most dependent smokers that require intensive support.

e. Providing advice and motivation from Level II trainers.

f. Following-up with a phone call and kept up-to-date with National Guidelines if patients do not attend weekly sessions.

2 STOP SMOKING! THE REASON WHY

People smoke for a number of reasons. Most smokers do it because they find it relieves stress and helps them relax. According to Preedy (2011) fashion models have shown that "the acceptance of smoking by females in order to maintain their weight needs to be investigated." Smoking can also be a source of support when things go wrong and can give a feeling of pleasure. These are all reasons why many people continue smoking once they've been diagnosed with cancer. Smoking is expensive, so quitting will save money. By smoking twenty cigarettes a day students can spend about £2,000 a year on cigarettes. Stopping means they will have more money to spend on other things. Evidence from inferential statistics[1] have led campaigners in Scotland wanting more to be done to protect children from adults who smoke. The Oxford Respiratory Medicine Library said that the NHS Stop Smoking service "is not clear where is the best place to deliver smoking cessation services. Of the 462,690 people under eighteen years of age setting a quit date in the quarter of year 2007 was fourteen thousand ." Within their publication Hill et al (2007) states that the "NHS Stop Smoking service is an important element of the Government strategy for tackling smoking." This may advise you on the benefits of stop-smoking in a specific situation or for a type of cancer. Having an understanding of how smoking affects your health may also motivate you to stop. Research shows that due to the chemicals in cigarettes this weakens the body's immunity and may help certain tumors to grow more quickly. Hill et al (2007) also confirmed that "the Department of Health recommends a multi-tiered approach, to providing support at the best possible way to reach more smokers, and gain the greatest reduction in smoking prevalence." The NHS Stop Smoking Services is free, local, and effective. They offer support that works and with determination and the students are up to four times more likely to quit smoking successfully if they go to the local NHS Stop Smoking service. Giving up smoking can cause nicotine withdrawal symptoms, which include cravings, headache, feeling irritable and not being able to sleep. The NHS Stop Smoking campaign provides an out reach service within the community, a place to walk-in for advice, on line advice, as well as stop smoking medicines on prescription which can help interested parties manage withdrawal symptoms.

3 WALK-IN CLINICS – THEIR OBJECTIVES

1. To target members of the community who feel they may need all the support they can get.

2. To inform an individual about Stop Smoking questionnaire which will determine how addicted they are, "one might argue that the only way of knowing whether someone is addicted is if they try to stop and the fail," West & Hardy (2006, page 11) The Cost Calculator is also introduced this shows how much can be saved.

3. To find the reasons and best way to help a student stop smoking if they want to and if they feel they are feel ready to do so.

4. To inform an individual about the consequences.

The Airdale and Bradford NHS services reports that "in England, one in every five deaths in adults over 35 is caused by smoking" and also "they may develop illness that may, according to the NHS get worse over time." It is obvious that the impetus behind the NHS lies with the findings of Alder et al (1999) which is "two thirds of the public would like to quit." The aim of the research is to prove that locally there are a variety of ways to help an individual quit smoking – and all of this lies within ones neighborhood, which makes it easier for everyone. Within each community it will be spelt out according to the Economics of Cancer Care publication that "reducing smoking is the most effective and immediate way of reducing mortality from cancer". The NHS is also certain of another factor and also according to Perkins et al (2007) "it should not be surprising that cigarette smoking alters brain function, is highly addictive, and is extremely difficult to stop." However, I am still reminded that the smoking cessation initiative is the most effective way for reducing the mortality of cancer.

Every cigarettes brand carries a government health warning therefore many are aware of the harmful effect it has upon their health. Chewing tobacco or smokeless smoking is very common in this day and age. Cordy (2001) addressed that "chewing tobacco or smokeless can cause lung cancer, even though they do not enter the body through the lungs." I also found if useful to mention that the author Spring (2009) remarked that "the number-one reason most people give for wanting to quit is to improve ones health." If individuals are aware of the pitfalls before hand that smoking brings, then, why do they engage in the first place? Are the reasons for smoking generally psychological?. People are seduced to try tobacco by the glamour of smoking in the movies and from advertisements. Addiction to nicotine makes it hard to quit once smoking has started. According to the leadership within the NHS campaign, addiction can be overcome in two weeks once the psychological reasons for smoking are eliminated.

4 GUIDANCE FROM THE DEPARTMENT OF HEALTH

The Department of Health is the organisation that draws attention to the core of an NHS stop smoking service: an NHS stop smoking service should meet a limited number of basic standards:

- weekly support must be offered for at least first four weeks out of quit attempt.
- four week follow-up should be carried out promptly.
- Only twelve weeks NRT (at max of two weeks prescribing) can be supplied using the Trusts P.G.D. (Patient Guide Direction) in association with pharmacists.
- stop smoking advisers must be appropriately trained.
- a minimum data set is needed for each client (including information about age and gender ethnicity and pregnancy status).
- Where possible smoking status of self-reported quitters should be confirmed by carbon monoxide (CO) validation.

Smoking is the number one preventable risk for ill health and inequalities. The local NHS Trust has decided to introduce an enhanced service for stop smoking advice under the new GP contract. Practices already contribute to the challenging the NHS Trust target. This enhanced service has been developed to support practices who offer stop smoking services in-house, and when appropriate, to support practices when referring patients to Level III specialist services. Practices offering these services in-house will need to allocate more resources to stop smoking and so this enhanced service has two levels that practices can opt to join thus ensuring the appropriate funding can be allocated.

Ongoing successful aims: the aims of this service are (both levels):

    a) To reduce smoking prevalence in practices' registered population.

    b) To raise awareness of the dangers of smoking and smoking related diseases.

    c) To enable those wishing to stop smoking to be given the appropriate help, information and support.

d) To increase the number of four week quitters as defined by the Russell Standard who access stop smoking services.

e) To target high risk groups who are smokers and refer them to the stop smoking service

5 THE BRADFORD CIY FIRE

Saturday 11th May 1985 became a national disaster for Bradford City. It was supposed to be a day of celebration for Bradford fans; their team had been promoted to the second division. Just before the kick off the Bradford City captain Peter Jackson had been presented with the Third Division Championship trophy. The match was being recorded for ITV televisions World of Sport, but as the drama unfolded, ITV's Saturday sports programme was interrupted. The whole nation was able to view the tragic events unfolding.

UK Fire Service Resources Group reported: "at 3.40pm with the score at 0-0 and only five minutes to go before half time a small fire was noticed three rows from the back of G block in the Valley Parade ground." Wikipedia mentioned that "most of the exits at the back were either locked or shut, and there were no stewards present to open them, but seven were either forced or found open". Stewards went on to request for fire fighting equipment, but within minutes flames became visible from under the stand so police and stewards started to evacuate people in the stand. UK Fire Service Resources Group believed that the fire started "when a spectator disposed of smoking materials, which fell through a damaged empty space beneath the seats of the main stand and onto a pile of rubbish that had accumulated beneath the stand for approximately 20 years." Ironically, the steel that the club said it intended to use to update the aging wooden roof the following Monday was lying in the car park behind the stand. The inquiry into the disaster, the Popplewell

Inquiry, led to the introduction of new legislation to improve safety at the UK's football grounds. One of the main outcomes of the inquiry was the banning of the construction of new wooden grandstands at UK sports grounds.

6 WHY FOCUS ON ANALYSIS OF DATA AND INTERPRETATION FINDINGS?

Apart from the Calculator Cost exercise there is unlikely to be too many data that might require elaborate statistical analysis of quantitative data. It is highly unlikely that the Stop Smoking campaign requires the necessity of inferential data analysis (i.e. conclusions that extend beyond the immediate data alone). Qualitative analysis (subjective judgment based on non quantifiable information) is expected to be more frequently used within the research than its quantitative counterpart. (i.e. the examination of measurable and verifiable data). Although there might be scope for a certain degree of quantifying some of the data, an overall non-quantifying method is likely to be used through the data analysis and interpretation process. I had the opportunity to sit-in and observe a number of sessions alongside a Stop Smoking advisor (level III). Some of the testimonies were predictable to the advisor, however I as the volunteer was intrigued by found out what lengths a patient would go to overcome this powerful addiction. At one of the sessions a smoker would state that they didn't smoke during the day or at home, but after a glass of wine. Because they drank every other night, they would end up smoking up to sixty cigarettes a week. They stress how their skin looked dull and they were beginning to get wrinkles around the mouth. It was then they realised it was seriously damaging their health. The Smoke Free Resource Centre suggests that "the first session should last for 90 minutes. The other six sessions will be an hour each." The co-ordinators are very friendly.

They will inform a smoker how the programme works, the aids available, such as patches and gum, and the 'quit date', which would be on the third session. Smokers are encouraged not to change they habits before then. The suggestion of joining a group is mentioned, this is according to the Department of Health "for people who don't want to give up alone." If one person is having a side effect, someone else will be going through the same thing. The charity Cancer Research stressed that during week two a smoker will be told that there are "4,000 chemicals in a cigarette" From my observation by week two a smoker was tested for carbon monoxide, a poisonous gas in tobacco smoke, which lowers oxygen in the bloodstream. You take a deep breath, then blow into a tube. If a smoker has not smoked for more than four days then the count would be pretty low. The advisor will also inform the smoker that included in the chemicals is carbon monoxide (CO), which hinders the oxygen in the red blood cells from functioning. The smoker is made aware that by not having a cigarette within 48 hours their CO reading will be as same as a non-smoker's reading, and it will remain that way until one decides to smoke again. By week three smokers will already be introduced to NRT (nicotine replacement therapy). The purpose of gums and patches is to take away most of the cravings. The use of NRT is highly recommended. They only last a maximum of four weeks. Within that time an individual can feel so much healthier. After week four an individual can loose the will power and decided to take a few cigarettes. "The support of the group made all the difference to me quitting" said Joseph P Weaver, winner of the 2002 American Cancer

Society Award (2012). He also states that "having a cigarette after you quit activates the brain's nicotine." He also went on to add "that's why you shouldn't even have a single puff."

There is an 0800 number to call to talk about why and how it will be so different the next time that situation arises. Two months is a long time to be without a cigarette, at that an individual will feel more in control and happier. The success depends upon whether they choose a support group or one-to-one sessions. It is made clear from the start that these sessions are free. The authors Wagner and Triggle (2003) touched on the area of what is a myth and what is a fact. But one of the classic myths is "it is easy to quit smoking because nicotine isn't that addictive." Wagner and Triggle say that "about two thirds of all young smokers say that want to stop." The leadership behind the Stop Smoking Campaign are faced with having to convince clients that the myths that lie behind the true effectiveness of the first day at the clinic. The Stop Smoking service continues to insist that their sessions are able to help an individual quit smoking.

7 MYTHS AND FACTS

The Myth	The Facts
1.Nicotine therapy causes cancer	This is wrong. Nicotine doesn't cause cancer. It's the other toxic chemicals in cigarettes, such as tar and carbon monoxide, which damage health. Nicotine replacement therapy gets nicotine into your body without the dangerous poisons.
2.Stop smoking treatments don't really work	Research suggests that nicotine replacement therapies and the prescription of stop smoking tablets (Champix and Zyban) can double and sometimes even triple the chances of successfully quitting. All stop smoking treatments work best when used as part of a programme that includes: • setting a quit date. • having a plan for dealing with things that make you reach for a cigarette. • getting support from a doctor or trained stop smoking adviser
3.It's dangerous to use more than one nicotine replacement product at a time	No, it isn't. In fact, using more than one product at a time – known as combination therapy – can be a good thing as it often

	increases your chances of success. A popular strategy is to use nicotine patches to reduce everyday cravings plus a nasal spray, gum, lozenges, inhalator or mouth spray for sudden cravings.
4.Champix will make me feel depressed	Champix has been linked with occasional reports of depression and even suicidal thoughts. However, it's not clear whether these side effects were due to the medicine or quitting smoking, and for most people it's perfectly safe. Talk with the doctor or NHS stop smoking adviser beforehand, especially if you have had another mental illness before. The occasional change in mood may be observed.. The GP should be informed if their is a change to an individual's condition.
5.Nicotine replacement therapy is expensive	NRT either free, or on prescription at a cost of £7.20 each week, from the local NHS Stop Smoking Service or the GP. That is up to a third cheaper than buying patches or gum from the pharmacy and is a lot cheaper than continuing to smoke until cravings for nicotine is no longer a necessity.

	Zyban and Champix are nicotine-free pills that is taken to reduce the craving for tobacco and help with withdrawal symptoms. In studies, Champix has been shown to work better than Zyban.
6.Stop smoking treatments will cure me	NRT and prescription medicines are not a miracle cure. They reduce cravings and withdrawal symptoms but they don't make them go away completely. There is still a need and effort placed into quitting but, as thousands of ex-smokers will testify, the medications really help.
7.I cannot use stop smoking treatments if I'm pregnant	If a woman is pregnant then it is a great time to quit as smoking is much more dangerous to the mother and the baby. The stop smoking adviser or midwife will talk about treatment options as the prescription tablets Champix and Zyban are not recommended in pregnancy. However, NRT products such as patches, gum, lozenges, microtabs, the inhalator and nasal sprays may be recommended if it is hard to quit.

8. I've had a heart attack so I cannot use NRT	Nicotine replacement therapy has been shown to be safe in most people with heart disease. However, because nicotine can increase the heart rate and blood pressure, it's a good idea to talk to a GP before using nicotine replacement products especially if a heart attack has been suffered in the past or one is experiencing irregular or rapid heartbeat.
9. Nicotine replacement products are as addictive as smoking	Most people using nicotine products do not become dependent on them. In fact, the biggest problem with NRT is that people don't use enough of it for long enough. The nicotine from patches, gum and so on is released into your system much more slowly and in a different way than nicotine from a cigarette. The body absorbs it more slowly and less reaches your brain.
10. I should not take the treatment Zyban because it causes seizures	There is a very small risk of having seizures (fits) when using Zyban. The risk increases if you've had seizures in the past. Therefore, it isn't recommended for anyone with a condition such as epilepsy.

I believe that the leadership behind the Stop Smoking campaign continues to be effective. NHS Stop Smoking Services have probably made a modest contribution to reducing inequalities in smoking prevalence to achieve government targets, because this requires both the development of more innovative cessation interventions for the most addictive smokers and action to ensure that other aspects of tobacco control policy make a larger contribution to inequality goals. The Department of Health Report (2007) state that the NHS stop smoking services "have continued to provide high-quality support to smokers who want to quit, this was higher in more deprived areas and concluded that this has made a positive contribution to the health inequalities."

8 HOW MUCH WILL YOU SAVE?

The National Non-Smoking day is usually on the 13th March. The leadership from the NHS Smoke Free campaign worked in conjunction with the Department of Health producing two initiatives that would determine how much one would save if they stopped smoking and also how quickly will their health improve. The Department of Health state that "thinking about the reasons to quit is a brilliant way to motivate oneself. There are many ways you can make improvements to your life and health by quitting." In order to find out how much can be saved the claimed that prices were "based on a packet of twenty cigarettes costing £7.09." National Statistics (April 2012).

5 cigarettes A Day @ (2 weeks)	10 cigarettes A Day @ (3 weeks)	15 cigarettes A Day @ (1 month)	20 Cigarettes A Day @ (6 months)	25 cigarettes A Day @ (1 year)
£700				
£600				
£500				
£400				
£300				
£200				25 a day
£100			20 a day	

	20 a day
£90	
£80	
£70	
£60	
£55	
£50	15 a day
£45	
£40	
£35	
£30	
£25	
£20	
£15	
£10	10 a day
£5	
£1	
£ Savings	

9 WHAT ARE THE BENEFITS?

The Department of Health recently drew attention to How Quickly
Will Your Health Improve and also its benefits. The complete
guidance can be found on the Department of Health website.

Quitting Span	Benefits
20 minutes	Blood pressure and pulse rate return to normal.
8 hours	Nicotine and Carbon monoxide levels in blood reduce by half and oxygen levels return to normal.
24 hours	Carbon monoxide eliminated from body. Lungs start to clear our mucus and other smoking debris.
48 hours	There is no nicotine in the body. Ability to taste and smell is greatly improved.
72 hours	Breathing becomes easier, bronchial tubes begin to relax and energy levels increase.
3-9 months	Coughs, wheezing and breathing problem improves as lung function is increased by up to 10%.
5 years	Risk of heart attack falls to about half that of a smoker.
10 years	Risk of lung cancer falls to half that of a smoker. Risk of heart attack falls to the same as someone who has never smoked.

10 CHURCH LEADERSHIP VIEWS ON SMOKING

If the qualitative research undertaken asks the reasons why, then my observations would be my approach for those reasons. This type of research is mainly subjective, i.e. what are people saying about the subject matter and what is it that I actually want to ascertain. The authors Alan and Bell (2007) stated the quantitative research criticise that "qualitative findings rely too much on the researcher's often un-systemic views about what is significant and important, and also upon the close personal relationships that the researcher frequently strikes up with the people studied." Alan & Bell (2007, page 423). As an observer I have come to the conclusion that it is the Christian's choice for doing if he or she wishes to smoke. The leadership within the Church leadership will see this as not being a good representative or a good witness. The Church leadership have their own way of helping an individual combat their smoking addiction; this is usually through prayer. It may even be recommended that they attend a Christian rehabilitation program. Unless the situation requires specialist medical attention; they will not necessarily work alongside the NHS. The leadership within the Church also believe that it is imperative that no one is left without access to health care. The organisation Health and Faith Connection state that "scientists have conducted research that has shown faith or spirituality has benefits in many areas such as cancer, hypertension, general health, heart disease, and other physical ailments as well as psychological, psychiatric and substance abuse problems." Faith and Health Connection, (2013). In the Bible smoking is seen as wasteful of time and of money because Christians are required to be good stewards of both.

11 THE BRITISH HEART FOUNDATION (BHF)

Ten million people in the UK still smoke. This was reported on Day Break TV (February 2013). A third of children hate the fact that their parents their parents still smoke. It could be because the parent's hair or clothes that smell of smoke. It could also be due to the fact that an innocent person who does not smoke can be more at risk of contracting cancer. Money and the saving money is the also a major reason why children feel that parents should quit; money could be better spent on a holiday abroad. Many parents are also spending more money on cigarettes rather than food. Smoking is an addiction. The future of an organisation that helps hundreds of thousands of people attempt to quit smoking has been assured. Prompted by a cut in statutory funding for No Smoking Day (NSD) and the fact quitting smoking is the single best thing you can do for your heart, NSD and the British Heart Foundation (BHF) have announced they intend to merge. The chief executive of No Smoking Day (2010), said: "No Smoking Day is one of the UK's longest-standing and most successful public health campaigns. But like many charities we've been severely affected by public sector cuts with 50 per cent of our total funding wiped out from next year. Fortunately, we've found a stable, long-term future for No Smoking Day."

Betty McBride, Director of Policy and Communications at the BHF, said: "By joining forces we can enhance the No Smoking Day campaign and extend its reach – helping more people to quit – as well as strengthening our policy and lobbying work. For both organisations, the opportunities posed by this merger were too good to miss." Because this provides secure funding for the campaign and a platform for growth, a rare opportunity in the current climate.

12 NO SMOKING DAY

This initiative supports thousands of local organisations across the UK, such as GP surgeries, schools, and employers, to host their own quit-smoking events on a single day. As well as promoting resources to help people quit, each organiser can highlight any or all of the range of health harms of smoking from heart disease and cancer through to the cosmetic effects on skin and teeth.

According to the official No Smoking Day campaign "more than 9 million UK adults still smoke, which equates to one in five. No Smoking Day is directly responsible for 250,000 people attempting to quit smoking each year. About 6,000 quit permanently, which means the campaign costs about £125 per person to help them quit for good. In contrast, it's estimated that smoking costs the NHS between £2.7bn and £5.2bn a year in the UK."

The purpose behind the NHS City and Hackney 2010 Smokefree Campaign was to allow smokers to meet their quitting goals through a new price promotion campaign run by both the NHS and Boots. The promotion was made available throughout January at the 3 Boots stores across Hackney (Dalston, Stamford Hill and Hackney). Members of the public who signed up for the in-store NHS stop smoking service had access to free stop smoking medication such as nicotine replacement therapy, as well as support. The smoking popularity in Hackney is 19%, based on data gathered from GPs. The campaign strategy follows research into the motivations of Hackney's smokers, which indicated that price promotion was an effective strategy. "Research shows that price can be a barrier to quitting for some smokers," said the then NHS City and Hackney Director of Public Health, "we hope that this month-long price promotion will make quitting that little bit easier, as well as introducing local residents and workers to the stop smoking support services available in the Hackney."

The overall aims of the price promotion campaign was to:

- Achieve a 50% success rate with those who sign-up to reach 4-week quit status.
- Increase the awareness that Boots UK provide local stop smoking services.
- Increase the number of people who try to quit smoking.
- Provide information about the dangers of smoking and what is available to help those who want to stop.

13 VIEWS ON TOBACCO CONTROL

A BBC news reportage (November 2010) announced that the Government had "still not committed to plain packaging for tobacco." Despite overwhelming support for the idea in its recent consultation. The report in the National Health Executive publication suggested that it was on its way, but was then restrained by the Prime Minister himself, who said "a decision has not been taken." Ailsa Rutter is the director of the award winning stop smoking service FRESH – Smoke Free North East. She informed the National Health Executive publication "the sooner that they can get on with this and implement it the better. Every day of delay, more children will be attracted to taking up smoking because of the glamorous glitzy packs. Implementing the measure would be fantastic and it would show real leadership from this Government around prioritising tobacco control." The director also went on to say that "is was early, although there is a feeling that there is compelling evidence that this will reduce the attractiveness to children and young people." It has been argued that the health warnings should be more prominent because adult smokers fool themselves into thinking that if they are smoking from a white silvery box that it is somehow less harmful than another type of cigarette. The director of the stop smoking service FRESH called it "a great opportunity for local government to make a real difference in addressing health inequalities within their communities." Harman (2001) stated that "tobacco smoking remains the single greatest cause of preventable illnesses and premature death in the UK." This is one of the major reasons why public health was transferred over to the local authorities. The National Health Executive (2013) believes in the responsibilities and powers of the local government and councils. Arguably the most important piece of legislation this century was the 2007 Public Smoking Ban, which has had better compliance than many had expected back then. The National Health Executive (2013) also commented on licensing tobacco retailers by stating that "there needs to be one for alcohol because anybody can sell tobacco." A number of councils have authority in terms of reducing youth access making sure retailers are compliant with the legislation.

14 THE INFLUENCE ON YOUNG PEOPLE

The teenagers of today are always keen to form an identity for themselves, especially if it means following or emulating those who influence society. Smoking is an identity and young people are influence by those around them, and prime figures under the media spot light. The Metro newspaper (March 2013) claimed that research shows that "the number of under-16s' who have taken up smoking rose 50,000 in a year. About 207,000 children aged 11-15 picked up the habit in 2011, while 27 per cent of uner-16s have smoked at least once, according to Cancer Research UK." They went on to say that "the charity called for plain packaging for tobacco in order to tackle the devastation caused by young people by the drug."

The Daily Mail (2010) reported that Dr Tony Jewell, chief medical officer for Wales, said that stopping people lighting up in their own homes would protect their children from the dangers of passive smoking. Opponents said the ban would be a breach individuals' right to privacy. However, Dr Jewell said it was "unfair for children to bear the brunt of other people's habits and it was time to make a change. As a society, creating such a measure is a powerful statement of intent about our commitment to the health of our children". He also argued that smokers know that smoking is a dangerous habit, but choose to ignore the facts". Smoking was banned publicly across Britain in April 2008. The Tobacco Manufacturers' Association's said Dr Jewell's proposals were 'a step too far and an unwarranted intrusion on individual freedom'. Whether it is in private vehicles, adults should be free to smoke, provided they do not light up or smoke in a way that would distract from safe driving. The Tobacco Manufacturers' Association's also went on to say that smokers should show due consideration for other occupants and dispose of cigarette ends responsibly in ashtrays. Wales is responsible for its own health policies under devolution. Smokers yesterday described the call as smacking of a 'Big Brother' state. If an individual smokes every day in front of the children but likes the occasional cigarette in front of the television while the children are in bed. Is it ridiculous for someone to be breaking the law in their own house? The Royal College of Physicians of London (2005) states that most deaths are caused by passive smoking at home.

15 THE CONCLUSION

NHS Stop Smoking Services have probably made a modest contribution to reducing inequalities in smoking prevalence to achieve government targets. This requires both the development of more innovative cessation interventions for the most addictive smokers and action to ensure that other aspects of tobacco control policy make a larger contribution to inequality goals. The Department of Health Report (2007) state that the NHS stop smoking services "have continued to provide high-quality support for smokers who want to quit, this was higher in more deprived areas and concluded that this has made a positive contribution to the health inequalities."

The Fire and Rescue service would also added, before emptying ashtrays make sure the contents are cold. Never smoke in bed. Before you go to bed make sure no cigarettes or pipes are still burning and never smoke in a chair if you feel you are going to doze off in it.

16 USEFUL REFERENCES

Bradford Football Fire:UK Fire Service (2013)

British Heart Foundation (2011)

Calculate the Cost: NHS Go Smoke Free

Children's Health for Dummies, Holland, K. & Jarvis, Dr. S.

Cigarettes could soon be sold in plain packets under
government plans: Metro Newspaper (2013)

Cognitive Behavioural Therapy for Smoking Cessation: Perkins, A.,
Conklin, C. A., & Levine, D. (2007)

Co-operative Doctor (2012): www.co-operativedoctor.co.uk/

Department of Health: Departmental Report 2007

Behaviour, Food and Nutrition: Preedy, V.R.

Make Cigarettes Plain Packaging: BBC Health (2010)

Nicotine is a Drug: Weaver, J.P. (2012)

Nicotine: Wagner H.L. and Triggle, D.J. (2003)

No Smoking Day (2012): http://smokingday.org.uk/press/

Public Health and Primary Care Partners in Population Health

Smoking Cessation - Oxford Respiratory Medicine Library

Smoking Cessation with Weight Gain Prevention: Spring, B.

Smoking and cancer, What's in a cigarette Cancer Research

"Smoking should be banned in Homes" Daily Mail online (2010)

Teaching Biblical Truths for Health and Wholeness Economics

The Royal College of Physicians of London (2005)

Tobacco - A Reference Handbook: Cordy, H. V. (2001)

Tobacco and Public Control: National Health Executive (2013)

What Are The Benefits: Department of Health (2013)

ABOUT THE AUTHOR

Jennifer has had an assorted career (including professional involvements in sports and as an actress) as well as spending a number of years working for the NHS.
She studied her degree (BA Hons in Leadership and Management) at Newham University College (NUC) and with the Open University.

Jennifer does not smoke. Her first publication is entitled *Words Pressed: A Short Biography*

www.ingramcontent.com/pod-product-compliance
Lightning Source LLC
Chambersburg PA
CBHW071015290526
45795CB00005B/1809